What You Should Know About Neuropathy

A Resilient Approach to Reversing
Neuropathy Naturally

By Dr. Rob Michaud DC, BS, BCN

Contents

About The Author

Dr. Rob Michaud is a Chiropractor in Kalamazoo, Michigan who is board certified from the American College of Physical Medicine (ACOPM) in treating Neuropathy. Originally from Saugatuck, Michigan, he and his wife, Dr. Chelsea Michaud, opened their Chiropractic clinic, Resilience Chiropractic in January of 2019 after graduating from Palmer College of Chiropractic in Florida. They are passionate about serving their community through providing natural and holistic options for treating various conditions that plague our society on a daily basis. While practicing at Resilience, Dr. Rob came across many practice members who were struggling with Neuropathy and being told that various medications were their only option, and/ or they would have to live with the condition. He became motivated to find another option for the neuropathy community, as he felt that the loss of hope they were given was simply unacceptable. Drs. Michaud truly believe that the body is a resilient organism, capable of far more than we are able to assess and give credit for. The natural treatment program discussed in this book was the result of his efforts.

CHAPTER 1

Viewing Health and Healthcare Through a Different Lens

As a practitioner, promoting holistic and natural options for the health of my patients is most important. However, the natural options often get overlooked and are not the standard recommendation in the western medical healthcare model. As you begin reading this book and we start this journey together, I encourage you to keep an open mind regarding overall health, take a step back and envision where you are currently and then where you want to be in the near future. This is not always an easy task, as we were all raised differently, come from different backgrounds, and have different experiences with utilizing natural solutions.

I didn't always view health in the way that I do now. It took trials, tribulations, frustrations, and wasted time for me to understand that my problems were not going to be solved by looking in the medicine cabinet. In my early twenties, I began the journey of trying to solve an episode of acute neck pain. I did what society has taught us; I went to my primary care doctor. Immediately, I was prescribed Gabapentin (which is an anticonvulsant mediation used primarily to treat seizures) and a few weekly steroid injections in the neck to treat my neck pain. It is often a common treatment protocol to prescribe Gabapentin and/or steroid injections for the pain if Ibuprofen or other non-steroidal anti-inflammatory drugs are not working. Similarly, Gabapentin is often a common drug used to "treat" neuropathy by blocking signals in the brain. In both of these scenarios, Gabapentin is altering the way that the brain perceives pain, but not directly addressing the root cause of the pain.

Just as Gabapentin is commonly prescribed in patients that are suffering from neuropathy, a few others are as well, such as Cymbalta, Lyrica, and opioid medication. In patients with neuropathy, the perception of pain is already altered. Some individuals feel no pain, some feel numbness, tingling, burning, can't sleep, can't walk, decreased balance, some cannot explain what it feels like at all. Although pain is annoying, it is an important sensation that signals that our bodies need help and that we may be in danger of hurting or injuring ourselves. This important bodily alarm system should not be masked by a drug. However, let's address the fact that patients with neuropathy usually have no other option because they cannot stand what they are feeling or lack there of; there are no other options available to them, so they chose to follow medical recommendations in hopes for a better future. This book will hopefully provide a new option for our readers and provide hope to those who have been told that they must learn to manage their neuropathy because there is no way around it.

Instead of searching for a band-aid approach to neuropathy, we should be working to find a way to heal and reverse this process naturally without the use of drugs or surgery. (Disclaimer: Please note, that I am not saying to stop taking those medications prescribed by your medical doctors; there is a time and place for medication and surgeries as some things cannot be avoided, but it should be treated as a last resort and for emergency situations. Please contact your medical doctor if you are looking to decrease or stop taking your medications altogether; there is a proper way to do so and should only be thought of as an option if your medical doctor is in agreement.) The United States has the best emergency care in the world, but when it comes to overall health, we are ranked last among highest performing nations. There needs to be a big change in the way that we view our health. Often, I hear from my patients that their doctors are informing them that neuropathy is a permanent condition that cannot be reversed. This is simply not true as we have hundreds of doctors across the country providing patient testimonials of how their neuropathy is in the process of or fully reversed. Myself, along with these doctors, are trying to change the trajectory of the standard of treatment for neuropathy. Of course, when it comes to neuropathy, there is a point of no return; when the nerve damage becomes so severe that it caused damage that is simply irreversible. Therefore, it is important to take action on your health now as naturally as possible, and not wait until we are forced to take action in the form of drugs and surgery.

As we reflect on what is truly important in our lives, we have to understand one important aspect: Our health is our greatest asset and without good health, we cannot enjoy the things that we love to do. Whether that is watching the sunrise or sunset everyday, playing with kids or grandkids, caring for your spouse and spending time with them, golfing, walking, enjoying retirement, vacations, and/or so much more, our lives are made brighter when our health is in good standing. By reading this book you are well on your way to taking the crucial next steps to healing your neuropathy, so let's dive in!

CHAPTER 2

America is in a Health Crisis

People tend to think of today's health crisis in the United States as a health *insurance* crisis. Fingers have been pointed at many parties for the current state of affairs:

- Government, for the lack of universal and affordable health insurance.
- Pharmaceutical companies, for the ever-increasing price of prescription drugs.
- Health care industry, for poor managed health care practices.
- Food industry, because lower income individuals are practically forced to purchase cheap, highly processed, unhealthy foods.

Although each of these parties has a hand in perpetuating the crisis, none of them is the true cause. The real reason behind the health care crisis is each individual's poor choices and lifestyle, mostly in the areas of food, exercise, and stress management. This leads to health-related issues like cancer, heart disease, metabolic syndrome, stroke, diabetes, and so much more.

Whether we like it or not, each one of us must take personal responsibility for our health. This means educating ourselves about the choices that will make a positive change for us and for those we love.

Biggest Health Issue Is Big Indeed

Perhaps the biggest health issue in the United States is obesity. In fact, it is at epidemic proportions. Among Americans age 20 and older, 154.7 million are overweight or obese.

18% of deaths in America are associated with obesity. These deaths stem primarily from type 2 diabetes, hypertension, heart disease, liver disease, cancer, dementia, and depression.

How Did the Obesity Problem Get So Big?

Early in the 20th century, the American diet was quite different from what it is today. If you could hop in a time machine and peek onto the shelves at the local store your grandparents shopped at, you would find produce, living plants, seeds, and grains. You might also find some home canned products. You would not find today's grocery store travesties:

- Hormone injected meats
- Processed foods
- Fast foods
- Junk foods

With these "modern" food choices comes a completely different diet – the SAD diet (Standard American Diet). The foods found in the SAD diet are completely out of balance.

1. An excessive amount of meat, fats, and sugar
2. Too few fruits and vegetables
3. Lack of nutrients in the food due to overcooking and processing

Incredibly, billions of dollars have been spent on various studies in a quest to find the causes and solutions for obesity. But the real answer is sitting in plain sight in homes across America: specifically, in the kitchens and on the couches.

The answer to the obesity crisis, and the health care crisis in general, is simple – returning to a more natural diet rich in fresh fruits and vegetables, while avoiding processed foods, and being active every day.

Trying to Make the Perfect Food Better

Food companies work tirelessly at making the perfect foods – fruits, vegetables and grains – better by refining them and processing them and adding chemicals to them. Ironically, all this tinkering has created an American diet that is deficient.

Processed foods make up a huge percentage of the American diet. These food products are loaded with extra salt, sugar, artificial flavors, preservatives, and other chemicals. These foods are also missing vital nutrients and vitamins that are stripped away during processing. This adding and subtracting from our food is a recipe for disaster.

Whole, natural foods are perfect foods. Eating a wide variety of fruits, vegetables, and grains gives your body everything it needs for good health. The SAD diet does not.

What It Is and What It Isn't

The Standard American Diet, sadly, is high in calories and low in nutrition. It consists of foods such as:

- Refined flour
- Refined sugar
- Refined cooking oil
- Soft drinks
- Coffee
- Margarine
- Distilled liquor

In order to be healthy, we need to replace low nutrient foods with high nutrient, non-processed foods, including:

- Vegetables
- Fruits
- Lean meat in moderation
- Fish

A healthy body needs a diet high in vitamins, minerals, enzymes and antioxidants. It's the best way to make sure your body can correctly digest food, absorb nutrients, regulate cell function, and keep your body fueled up.

When your body doesn't have the nutrients it needs, the aging process speeds up. Aging doesn't just mean gray hair and wrinkles – we are talking about all the diseases associated with aging, such as:

- Coronary Heart Disease (CHD): About 600,000 people die of heart disease in the United States every year–that's 1 in every 4 deaths.

- Coronary heart disease alone costs the United States $108.9 billion each year.

- Stroke: In 2009, stroke caused 1 of every 19 deaths in the United States. On average, every 40 seconds, someone in the United States has a stroke. Every four minutes, someone dies from a stroke.

- High Blood Pressure: Based on data from 2007 to 2010, about 78 million people in the United States age 20 and older have high blood pressure.

- Cancer: In 2012, there were approximately 13.7 million Americans with a history of cancer. Some of these men and women were cancer-free and others still had evidence of cancer and could be undergoing treatment. In 2013, there were expected to be 1,660,290 new cancer cases.

- Diabetes: Data from the 2011 National Diabetes Fact Sheet states that 25.8 million people in the United States has diabetes. 1.9 million new adult cases of diabetes were diagnosed in 2010. An update in 2013 states that the total cost of diagnosed diabetes in the United States in 2012 was $245 billion.

- Osteoporosis: More than 40 million Americans are estimated to already have this disease.

The United States is reported to spend over eight thousand dollars per person on healthcare. It is hard to believe that there are people dying of an inadequate diet in the United States when there is a surplus of food, but it's true. And there appears to be little hope of reversing the trend.

The World Health Organization (WHO) ranked the U.S. number one in health care spending. But even with all this spending, the U.S. ranked 72 in overall health – lower than many Third World countries.

The Real Answer

People like to think that modern medicine is the answer to the health care crisis. But experts in the field of medicine realize that despite the use of advanced technology, there has been no decline in the health crisis.

The real answer does not rely on the curing of disease, but in the prevention of it. And one of the best ways to prevent disease is living a healthy lifestyle. For many people, understanding what constitutes a healthy lifestyle is daunting. Other people know exactly what "healthy living" means, but they are not willing to commit to making the necessary lifestyle changes. Committing to choices like these simply sounds like too much of a hassle:

1. Eat well – Kick the SAD diet out of your life and replace it with a diet filled with fresh fruits and vegetables, whole grains (limited), lean meats, healthy fats, and fish.
2. Exercise well – Exercising just 30 minutes three times per week will promote heart health, help you lose weight by increasing your metabolism, build strong bones, and boost your immune system.

3. Sleep well – Most cell repairs and memory assimilation happen during sleep. Most people need seven to eight hours of sleep each night in order to function at their best.

4. Live well – Believe it or not, kindness and love, as well as having a set of principles to guide your life, will help you to be healthier and live longer.

5. Optimal Nervous System Health – Everything that goes on in our body begins with the nervous system. Ridding your body of blockages in the nervous system, known as subluxations, can help you reach your full potential.

The burden of achieving good health falls squarely on your own shoulders. You cannot rely on others to watch out for your health. You cannot find good health at the doctor's office or in the pharmacy. You can't find it in the junk food aisles of the grocery store or in fast food restaurants. Good health can only be found when you commit to a healthy lifestyle.

By taking care of your body now, learning everything you can to make good choices, and finding practitioners that promote the prevention of disease, you will be well on your way to a healthier you.

CHAPTER 3

Crisis Care vs. Longevity Focus

Modern medicine is crisis-focused. It's one of the things that allows the average American to burn the candle at both ends for a few decades, have a little open heart surgery to keep the old ticker chugging along, and skid into a late retirement exhausted, disabled, and broke.

Think about it.

Are you motivated to be well right now, or will you be far more motivated to be well when you get sick and your life is taken away from you? Sadly, we only tend to find our motivation when something goes wrong. It's far easier to choose cheeseburgers and couch time over healthier choices... until all those bad choices finally create a disaster for our health.

That's the real cause of the vast majority of diseases we are dealing with today: lifestyle choices. We should be motivated every day to live a lifestyle that allows us to thrive, maintain, and enjoy a fantastic quality of life. And that's what the wellness movement is all about: seeking wellness instead of seeking cures, each and every day. There is no medication, special lotion, surgery, and injection that re-gains our health back.

Modern medicine runs on the philosophy that aging is the decline phase of life. We are born, we live, we get sick, and we die. But it doesn't have to be that way! There's the first mindset switch we need to make. Instead of thinking of our bodies as vessels destined and designed for deterioration and disease, think of it as being meant for continuous progress. Yes, we will all age, and we will all eventually die. But how would the rest of your life be different if you decided to live up to your physical potential from here on out?

What Is Wellness Care?

More and more people are coming to realize that focusing on their wellness could allow them to live healthier, longer lives. They are demanding that their health care providers work with them on wellness plans that prevent, rather than cure, diseases and pain. There is evidence of this shift all around us:

- Organic and local foods are becoming the preferred produce option in America, and around the world. The USDA's National Farmers Market Directory's listings have increased by more than 61% since 2008.
- The Veterans Administration has committed to implementing alternative therapies to help veterans deal with pain and avoid possible opioid painkiller addictions.
- According to Harvard Medical School, Americans make about 425 million visits to holistic health care providers each year.
- A 2011 Gallup poll showed that half of Americans take vitamins every day.

Part of the wellness revolution has been a shift in the relationship between primary care doctors and patients. By and large, the public no longer chooses to take their doctor's advice as the final word on certain health concerns. We are far more likely today to ask questions, seek second opinions, and research alternative treatments. The patient, rather than the doctor, is now the decision-maker when the patient's wellness is concerned.

What IS Modern Medicine Good For?

Make no mistake: modern medicine still plays an important role in our health care system. And the more open and receptive your primary care physician is to discuss your wellness care, the more of a partner role he or she can play in your ongoing health.

The modern view on health care places all health-related concepts and activities into three categories:

1. Self Care – this includes the choices you make every day about diet, exercise, stress management, and the like.

2. Health Care – this is all of the things you seek help for in order to maintain good health, such as seeking wellness providers, getting educated on fitness and exercise, and taking part in wellness programs physicians are offering.

3. Crisis Care – this is the care we obtain when a disaster strikes; when we get sick or injured, we go to the doctor to help us fix what we cannot handle on our own.

Self care and health care are intended to prevent the need for crisis care. However, choosing to stop smoking will not prevent you from getting into a car accident. There are sure-fire ways to prevent cancer, heart attacks, or other conditions, but of course there are occurrences were serious illnesses, broken bones, failing organs - situations such as these are the rightful domain of crisis care.

A Crash Course in How to Get Well

America's current health care system promotes drugs and surgery above all else – including prevention. Each year, America spends $3 billion on prescription medications and $2 trillion on crisis care. The first tragedy of this situation is that despite all that spending, America is still getting sicker and sicker. The second tragedy is that most of the illnesses for which we seek crisis care are completely preventable.

Chances are, there are about a hundred lifestyle choices you could improve upon. Here are a few simple suggestions to get you back on track:

- Get regular, moderate exercise
- Stay well hydrated
- Eat a plant-based, nutrient-dense diet
- Get adequate sleep
- Quit smoking and any other drug habits
- Enjoy moderate alcohol intake at the most
- Find healthy ways to deal with stress
- Seek activities and people that boost your mood
- Bring aboard health care practitioners you trust to help you feel well

In later chapters, we will dig into many of these topics in more detail. Suffice it to say that people tend to feel stressed and conflicted when making these lifestyle shifts. It's just so much easier to give in to our desires... to be lazy and not hit the gym... to order the cheeseburger because it's on the happy hour menu but the salad isn't... to quit smoking, maybe next week.

All of those choices we make every day seem insignificant in the moment. But it all adds up. In ten, twenty, thirty years from now, will you regret your lifestyle choices? What it all comes down to is this – how can you improve your current level of functioning?

CHAPTER 4

Peripheral Neuropathy and What You Need to Know

What is Peripheral Neuropathy? It helps to break the term down and look at each individual word. **Neuropathy** refers to pain that is caused by nerve damage. The **peripheral** part of the term refers to the peripheral nervous system – that's all of the nerves in your body that radiate out from your spinal cord. So peripheral neuropathy is typically presented as pain and tingling caused by nerve damage in the extremities.

The most common areas affected by peripheral neuropathy are the nerves in the extremities, like your arms, hands, legs, and feet. People with peripheral neuropathy generally describe the pain as stabbing, tingling, numbness, burning, or icy coldness. Many of these patients also report some weakness in the affected area.

Neuropathy of the small fiber nerves reduces sensation and can cause the patient not to be able to feel cuts, burns, punctures, or blisters on the skin. Reduced sensation in the feet can cause car accidents when people fail to sense whether they are pressing the gas pedal or the brake, or they may not be able to regulate the pressure they apply to a pedal.

Neuropathy of the large fiber nerves in the legs can cause loss of balance and coordination. This type of neuropathy causes thousands of falls every year. A fall puts the patient at risk for hip fractures, head traumas, and other serious injuries.

Typically, an EMG (Electromyogram) will be ordered if any of these symptoms are present. Most likely the test results will come back normal. The problem with this is it is testing for damage to muscles innervated the motor nerves (nerves that initiate movement and control muscles), it does not test for the sensory portion of nerves, which would correctly correlate with neuropathy sensory symptoms. In this way, an EMG would give us valuable information, just not fully the information we would need which would leave us thinking that the problem is not as severe as in may in fact be.

In addition to the extremities, other parts of the body can be affected by neuropathy; for example, the peripheral nervous system also controls your vital organs. Damage to the associated nerves can cause heartburn, indigestion, difficulty swallowing, constipation, and many other problems.

What Causes Peripheral Neuropathy?

Instead of delving into the hundreds of specific causes there are for peripheral neuropathy, we will break them down into three general categories.

1. **Circulation related peripheral neuropathy** is most often experienced by people with diabetes, but anyone with reduced blood circulation is at risk. When the small blood vessels surrounding the nerves die off, the

nerves are deprived of nourishment and will also eventually die. The damaged nerves are the source of the pain and tingling.

Over 50% of diabetics develop some form of neuropathy (Mayo Clinic). Peripheral neuropathy is also the top cause of amputations for diabetics.

2. **Toxicity related peripheral neuropathy** can be caused by any sort of exposure to toxins. The two causes we typically focus on are chemotherapy drugs and statins.

   a. **Chemotherapy-induced peripheral neuropathy** is a side effect reported by many cancer patients. Some chemotherapy drugs are more likely to cause neuropathy than others. Patients who are on a more frequent treatment schedule are also more likely to experience neuropathy.

   b. **Statin-induced peripheral neuropathy** is caused by the use of drugs that doctors prescribe to reduce fats, including tri- glycerides and cholesterol, in the blood.

Instead of prescribing changes in diet and exercise habits to fix the root cause of the cholesterol problem, it is far easier (and more profitable) for a doctor to prescribe a statin.

3. **Trauma induced peripheral neuropathy** is caused by events like car accidents, falls, or athletic injuries. Any of these events can cause damage to the peripheral nerves. Wearing a cast, walking with crutches, or frequent repetitive motions can also damage nerves. (Mayo Clinic)

One important fact to realize is that regardless of the cause of peripheral neuropathy, the damage is the same under a microscope. The techniques for rebuilding the nerves does not change.

How Do You Treat Peripheral Neuropathy?

Medical doctors routinely tell their patients that nerves cannot regenerate themselves, but it's simply not true! Several treatments have been proven to stimulate the growth of the nerve endings and the blood vessels that nourish them.

If the symptoms are caused by a treatable underlying condition, it is almost always possible to reverse the neuropathy. While medications can reduce the pain associated with peripheral neuropathy, painkillers do nothing to repair or reverse the damage to the nerves and blood vessels. Getting to the root cause of the neuropathy and taking steps to reverse the damage is the only effective and long-lasting method of treatment.

The end goal in treating peripheral neuropathy is to remove blockage so that the nerves can function properly and send and receive messages with the brain. The best way to achieve this is with a comprehensive treatment plan. That's why we use several methods concurrently to treat our peripheral neuropathy patients.

Peripheral Neuropathy Treatment Options

Low Level Light Therapy (LLLT) – LLLT uses low-power lasers or infrared light-emitting diodes to promote nerve growth, reduce pain, improve immune response, accelerate healing of wounds and fractures, increase collagen and DNA production, and promote fibroblast activity.

Vibration Therapy – Vibration therapy is recommended to increase balance and mobility, bone density, and range of motion. It also increases blood flow by 15 times. During vibration therapy, patients sit or stand on a vibrating platform that causes their muscles to contract, increase circulation, as well as nerve stimulation.

ReBuilder System – Uses electrical stimulation of the muscles to improve blood flow and normalize deficits in nerve conduction velocity. The ReBuilder System is trusted by all four Cancer Treatment Centers of America locations to alleviate chemotherapy-induced peripheral neuropathy. Most of their cancer patients who use the Re-Builder System have reduced or stopped taking their pain medicine, as they report drastically reduced pain in their extremities after treatments.

Spinal Decompression - When peripheral neuropathy has resulted from an accident or injury that resulted in compressed discs or vertebrae, spinal decompression can provide relief. Spinal decompression is a chiropractic technique that uses traction to take the pressure off the discs and allow the discs to move back into place. It also stimulates blood flow, which produces a healing response.

Traditional chiropractic therapy is used by millions of people to adjust misaligned vertebrae. Regular chiropractic care allows signals to flow between the brain, spinal cord, and nerves. Since chiropractic adjustments promote nervous system function, it should be considered an integral part of any peripheral neuropathy treatment plan. More importantly with neuropathy, chiropractic is used to get the feet and hands more mobile as the neuropathy has created stiffness and mobility problems.

Each intricate part of our program is equally important. Each one relies on the other to do its job. There are a lot of treatments out there that get new blood to the areas temporarily. We know them all; our goal is to repair neuropathy permanently.

These treatment methods will be discussed in more detail in the following chapters.

What Else Can I Do to Reduce My Pain?

There are additional components of a full peripheral neuropathy treatment plan that cannot be controlled in the clinic setting. While we provide our patients with the resources to make the right choices for themselves, it is solely up to them how closely they follow these guidelines.

Nutrition – Committing to dietary changes that reduce inflammation in the body can make a tremendous difference in peripheral neuropathy symptoms. Basically, an anti-inflammatory diet promotes foods that inhibit inflammation (fruits, vegetables, lean omega-3 rich foods) and limits the intake of foods that promote inflammation (sugars, starches, omega-6 foods).

Supplements – Natural Nitric Oxide Boosters is an intricate part of treating peripheral neuropathy. In the following chapters, we will take a closer look at the peripheral neuropathy treatment options we offer in our clinic.

CHAPTER 5

Low Level Light Therapy – Can It Help You?

Since lasers were invented in the 1960's, medical professionals have discovered numerous applications for lasers to improve people's health. Ophthalmologists, dermatologists, and surgeons quickly found lasers to be useful in treating their patients. Low level light therapy (LLLT) is in its fourth decade of use as a method of treating sprains, back and neck pain, arthritis, ulcers, and more.

Looking to the future, studies are currently being conducted to test out LLLT's effectiveness in treating sperm mobility, spinal cord injuries, stroke victims, Parkinson's patients, and Alzheimer's disease.

How Does LLLT Work?

Think back to your high school biology class. You may recall that plants use a process called photosynthesis to produce energy. The plant changes that energy into ATP, which is the fuel stored and used by all cells in all living things – plants and animals alike. LLLT stimulates the production of enzyme cytochrome c oxidase, which, like sunlight for plants, produces ATP. With more fuel being produced, cells have more energy to repair themselves. Currently, numerous studies being conducted around the world are proving that LLLT can help the body regenerate its own tissues, including spinal cord and nerve tissues. The therapy also holds promise for restoring eyesight, reversing numerous neurological diseases, and stroke recovery.

What Else Could LLLT Treat in the Future?

Fibromyalgia is a condition that causes the brain to process pain abnormally, resulting in chronic, widespread pain and chronic fatigue. This condition affects millions of Americans and has been poorly understood and under-diagnosed, resulting in billions of dollars in cost to our health care system.

Fibromyalgia is primarily treated with medications; side effects often make the patient's symptoms even worse. But studies have already shown that LLLT helps to treat the pain and swelling of fibromyalgia.

Parkinson's Disease belongs to a group of conditions called motor system disorders, which are the result of the loss of dopamine-producing brain cells. The four primary symptoms of Parkinson's disease are tremors in the arms, legs, jaw, and face; stiffness of the limbs and trunk; slowness of movement; and impaired balance and coordination.

Many scientists think that one of the malfunctioning systems in Parkinson's disease is located in the mitochondria. These are the cellular systems/organelles that produce ATP, the energy for all the other systems of the body. They also help to detoxify the brain and body by regulating the free radicals circulating in the system.

A study by the UVA Morris K. Udall Parkinson's Research Center of Excellence showed that a single, brief treatment of LLLT increased the movement of the mitochondria in neuron cells to be similar to the level of movement in disease-free, age-matched control groups.

Muscle regeneration is another area where LLLT holds great promise. LLLT has been shown to increase cellular function and regeneration, including cells that create muscle tissue. Studies are being conducted to determine if heart muscles can be regenerated using LLLT.

Medical doctors are taught that heart muscle does not regenerate. Therefore, when someone has a heart attack, doctors tell patients that the muscle that died in the attack is gone for good. However, new research shows that heart muscle can and does regenerate itself. This finding opens up new possibilities of regenerating heart muscle after a heart attack with LLLT, thereby preventing a host of complications including heart failure.

Weight loss might sound like a stretch when you think of the possibilities of LLLT treatment, but it is already being used to help patients achieve their goals. Laser light easily penetrates through layers of skin to activate healing responses within cells and to stimulate nerve endings to produce endorphins. Endorphins, such as serotonin, are produced normally by your body and are nature's natural mood lifter and help prevent you from feeling anxious or moody.

The LLLT therapy of specific points on the body helps to reduce the desire to eat, providing a natural satiation without food. The laser also helps balance organ and glandular functions that regulate weight. Incredibly, LLLT is used in a very similar way to relieve the withdrawal symptoms of quitting smoking!

Diabetic ulcers are one of the many health risks associated with uncontrolled diabetes. Diabetic ulcers are extremely hard to cure. Due to artery abnormalities, diabetic neuropathy, and delayed wound healing, infection or gangrene of the extremities is relatively common.

Wound healing is usually taken care of efficiently by a healthy body. But diabetes is a disorder that impedes normal steps of the wound healing process. Common treatments - skin grafts, moist wound therapy, and negative pressure wound therapy – almost never work completely.

LLLT is a new treatment option for diabetic ulcers that is showing great promise. Unlike other therapies, LLLT has no side effects. In one case study, a man with a diabetic ulcer was treated for a total of 16 sessions of low-intensity laser therapy over a four-week period. During this time, the ulcer healed completely. During a follow-up period of nine months, there was no recurrence of the ulcer.

What Role Does LLLT Play in Treating Peripheral Neuropathy?

Because LLLT stimulates cellular regeneration, it plays a vital role in a complete treatment plan for peripheral neuropathy patients. LLLT helps damaged nerves and their surrounding blood vessels regrow, gradually improving sensation and function for the patient. There are currently no drugs on the market that can help the body heal itself in such a way. Plus, unlike virtually all medications, there are absolutely no side effects associated with LLLT. The area may feel warm or tingly during the treatment, but there are no other reported physical sensations from LLLT patients.

If determined necessary for your specific case, LLLT may be added to your comprehensive treatment plan on your hands, feet, or both for a specified amount of time in order to empower your body for regeneration.

CHAPTER 6

Electrotherapy for Neuropathy Pain Relief and Nerve Re-Education

Right off the bat, let's get one thing out of the way: this is nothing like the horrifying practice of electroshock therapy that was used in asylums decades ago. And on the other hand, it's more exciting than the electrolysis procedure that can get rid of unwanted body hair.

Electrotherapy is a pain management technique where small electrical currents stimulate nerves and muscles to release pain-killing chemicals such as endorphins, and prevents pain signals from being transmitted to the brain. Electrotherapy also improves nerve function by gently opening up the nerve pathways. It does not hurt your muscles or nerves, and it does not burn your skin. In our office, we rely on the ReBuilder System for patients seeking treatment for peripheral neuropathy. This technology is much different than a TENS unit. TENS units can actually make neuropathy worse over time.

ReBuilder is an FDA-approved device that was designed specifically to treat the pain, burning, numbness, and tingling associated with peripheral neuropathy. In fact, all of the Cancer Treatment Centers of America use ReBuilder to alleviate their patients' chemotherapy-induced neuropathy.

What Are the Benefits of ReBuilder Treatment?

Daily, thirty minute ReBuilder treatments in your home may significantly reduce the amount of pain medications needed to deal with an acute pain syndrome. It has also been used to effectively treat functional problems such as drop foot. The effects of this treatment method are cumulative, meaning that the longer you continue to use it, the better the results you will see.

ReBuilder also increases blood flow, strengthens muscles, and improves the transmission of signals within the nervous system. And when patients experience less pain at night, they tend to get a better night's sleep. This allows them to function better during the daytime and promotes cellular repair and regeneration during their restful hours.

How Do I Use ReBuilder at Home?

You will place small adhesive pads in a supplied footbath, or place the effected areas on specific pads in order to deliver electrical current. Your healthcare provider will help you determine where the pads should be placed for best results. The vast majority of patients, marked improvement in pain, function, and mobility occurs within just a few electrotherapy treatments.

How Does it Work?

All you have to do is put on the pads or garments, turn on the system, and sit back so that the device can do its job. ReBuilder is an "intelligent" system, in that it analyzes the nerves 7.83 times per second, determines the correct amount of electrical signal, and then delivers it to the target area.

The electrical current opens up the nerve pathways and promotes good signal conduction. During treatment, you may feel your muscles contract and relax – this is normal. As you progress through more and more treatments, your condition will improve and the need for electrotherapy is reduced. Throughout the treatment period, the ReBuilder will alter the amount of signal it delivers based on the condition of your nerves.

Whether your peripheral neuropathy is a side effect of statin drugs, chemotherapy treatment, diabetes, or another source, ReBuilder can help restore function and sensation to your peripheral nervous system.

Why Is ReBuilder the Electrotherapy System of Choice?

Since ReBuilder hit the market in the mid 1980's, it has helped millions of patients repair their pain points from the inside out with no drugs, no surgery, and virtually no side effects. When you have dealt with problems like shortness of breath, memory loss, constipation, sleeplessness, and dizziness while on pain medications, the idea of treating the root cause of the pain and eliminating drugs from your daily routine often seems like nothing more than a fantasy. But it's totally possible – perhaps within a week or two – with electrotherapy.

Another benefit of the ReBuilder System is that it shuts off automatically when the treatment time is up. This prevents possible injury, should the patient fall asleep during treatment. ReBuilder also comes with a lifetime warranty.

But the real reason we use ReBuilder for our peripheral neuropathy patients is simple: we have seen the results first-hand. Almost all of our patients who use ReBuilder report feeling less numbness, pain, and tingling in the treated area. With blood flow and nerve function restored, patients become more mobile and stop relying on painkillers to get through the day.

Is ReBuilder Right for Me?

In our clinic, we are all about helping our patients heal from the inside out, without medications or surgery. We use several modalities at once to treat our patients who are suffering from peripheral neuropathy because we believe in a broad-spectrum approach to treating chronic pain. All of the techniques we combine for neuropathy treatment are focused on improving nerve function and regeneration, as well as promoting blood flow.

Our neuropathy patients come to us in the midst of a very difficult period in their lives. They may be going through chemotherapy treatment; maybe they are failing to recover from an automobile accident; they could also be suffering from diabetes-induced neuropathy. While the causes of their pain are different, we use similar methods to treat them all. Electrotherapy is one important treatment method that they all have in common.

Thousands of doctors in all types of practices prescribe the ReBuilder System for their patients. All four Cancer Treatment Centers of America offer it to their patients who are undergoing chemotherapy. And as a matter of fact, using ReBuilder *before* starting treatment can be an effective preventative measure against developing peripheral neuropathy in the first place.

If you are suffering from the effects of peripheral neuropathy, there is an excellent chance that ReBuilder can help. The ReBuilder is only a piece of the puzzle in our innovative program. We strongly believe that a more complete approach to Neuropathy Reversal is a smarter plan of action. That's why we prescribe electrotherapy, low level light therapy, chiropractic, Nutrition, and vibration therapy to our patients who are struggling to get their pain under control and live an active life like they desire.

CHAPTER 7

Vibration Therapy and the Benefits

Health care providers, physical therapists, chiropractors, and personal trainers use whole body vibration therapy (WBVT), for a surprisingly wide range of purposes. Specifically, vibration therapy is great for:

- Increasing muscle endurance, coordination, and strength
- Better circulation of lymph fluid and blood for better healing, energy, and overall health
- Improving nerve activity
- Boosting bone density and fighting off osteoporosis

For our patients with peripheral neuropathy, vibration therapy reduces their pain, increases circulation, improves strength and flexibility, and increases energy, mobility, and balance. We achieve these results without drugs or invasive surgery.

A recent study showed that patients with diabetic peripheral neuropathy (DPN) specifically have much to gain from vibration therapy. Study participants were observed to determine how effective whole body vibration therapy really is in treating pain associated with DPN. The study's participants received three whole body vibration treatments per week for a month. Each session consisted of four rounds of three minutes of vibration. The study's results demonstrated significant pain reduction overall, and no side-effects were observed during the study.

WBVT allows individuals to experience less pain without invasive surgery, and usually reduces or even eliminates the need for pain medication. The high-frequency vertical vibrations produced by the device assist in increasing circulation, rebuilding muscle tissue, improving range of motion, and reducing pain and stress. But the benefits go even further beyond getting off pain medications. Patients are likely to see far fewer serious injuries and infections due to increased sensation and better coordination. And diabetics in particular will be at lower risk of limb amputation due to reduced infection rates.

How Does WBVT Work?

Vibration therapy devices come in a range of forms. There are vibrating foot platforms that treat just peripheral neuropathy of the feet. Some practitioners use hand-held devices to target very specific areas of the body and fully customize the length and duration of treatment. Other health care providers prefer vibrating chairs or platforms that patients may sit or stand on for a full-body treatment. Either way, the high frequency vibration is an effective and safe treatment for the area(s) of the body affected by neuropathy.

Vibration therapy stimulates a patient's muscles to rapidly contract. Frequent tightening of a muscle will build and strengthen the muscle tissue, even when it's performed for small bits of time. As the muscle builds, its need for blood also grows. This is what stimulates blood vessels to grow and keep fueling the muscles with the nutrients they need during and after vibration therapy.

It's important to note that while traditional exercise is difficult and often uncomfortable for many patients dealing with chronic pain, vibration therapy cuts these complications out of the equation. When people have reduced sensation in their feet and hands, it can be downright dangerous to pick up free weights or hop onto a treadmill. But vibration therapy allows the patient to sit down throughout the "workout," even though muscles are being strengthened the entire time.

When the muscles are pushed and exerted in specific ways, the nerves can be stimulated to regrow their neural pathways and even repair or rebuild the damaged nerves.

An added bonus of vibration therapy is that it stimulates the release of osteoblasts from the nuclei in bone cells. Osteoblasts are what make it possible for bones to grow stronger by creating new bone cells.

All of these facts combined means that vibration therapy patients will regain sensation, strength, and stamina. Over time, the little things in life that used to be exhausting will become far easier. Eventually, patients get back to more normal routines and introduce regular moderate exercise to their daily calendars. It is truly an eye-opening experience to lose full use of parts of your body, and then gain it back again. Your priorities and your perspective will never be the same.

Is There Anybody Who Should NOT Experience WBVT?

Certain patients should not participate in vibration therapy, including patients with epilepsy, severe vertigo, or a detached retina. Also, if you are pregnant, vibration therapy is probably not safe for you.

For the rest of our patients who may benefit from it, we recommend vibration therapy, which we also provide in our office. Vibration therapy treatments usually last no more than about 15 minutes. But the key to effectively treating many conditions, including peripheral neuropathy, is to approach it with several different modalities. That's why we never treat a peripheral neuropathy patient with just vibration therapy.

Our peripheral neuropathy patients utilize low-level light therapy, electrical stimulation, nutritional protocols, neurologically-based chiropractic care, vibration therapy and soft tissue treatments, all as a well rounded approach to their condition. We go at these pain-related conditions with everything we've got, because patient comfort, health, and satisfaction is paramount. We know that this multi-pronged approach is the best way to get people off painkillers and back on their feet. That's why we also continuously counsel our patients about the importance of proper hydration and diet. You really are what you eat, so it's crucial to fuel your body with healthy, high-quality foods that will promote growth, healing, and wellness in every cell of your body. Continue on to the next chapter to learn more about the role good nutrition plays in your recovery from peripheral neuropathy.

CHAPTER 8

Good Health Starts with Good Nutrition

Getting regular exercise, dealing with stress in healthy ways, and eating a diet rich in plant-based whole foods is a great start toward achieving good health. But no matter how well you stick to these tips, you are always at risk for your body to be damaged at the cellular level. Environmental factors play a huge part in this damage by introducing free radicals into our bodies.

What Are Free Radicals?

Free radicals form in the human body when an electron in an atom becomes unpaired and searches for another electron to pair with. It may sound like an insignificant event, but this search for another unpaired atom causes damage to our cells and a chain reaction of more free radical creation.

Daily life exposes us to free radicals all the time, from the foods we eat and the air we breathe. Free radicals cause illness and contribute to the aging process. They have a negative impact on how we look and feel. Free radicals occur in everyday life but are made worse by:

- Eating a diet full of processed foods and produce treated with chemicals
- Smoking
- Using drugs
- Failure to deal correctly with stress
- Excessive sun exposure
- Pollution

Free radical damage can lead to:

- Cancer
- Heart Disease
- Diabetes

- Arthritis
- Autoimmune Diseases

One thing we can do to fight free radicals is to get more antioxidants in our diets. Antioxidants are vitamins, minerals, and other nutrients that protect the body and fight off free radicals. They give free radicals an electron to pair with before the stray electrons can damage our cells. Some examples of antioxidants are beta carotene, vitamin C, and vitamin E. These vitamins help strengthen the immune system, too. Plus, they're readily available in many plant-based foods which we should consume more of, anyway!

Beta Carotene

Beta carotene is one of a group of red, orange, and yellow pigments called carotenoids. Beta carotene and other carotenoids provide approximately 50% of the vitamin A needed in our daily diet.

Beta carotene is a substance the body converts into vitamin A. It's a powerful antioxidant that also helps protect the cells and boost the immune system. Sources of this important nutrient include:

- Carrots
- Pumpkins
- Sweet potatoes
- Spinach
- Collards
- Kale
- Turnip greens
- Beet greens
- Winter squash
- Cabbage

If you would rather get your vitamin A straight-up instead of through the beta carotene conversion, eat more:

- Beef
- Broccoli
- Cantaloupe
- Apricots
- Liver
- Milk
- Butter

- Cheese
- Whole eggs

Vitamin C

When your mom told you to drink orange juice to get over a cold faster, she was right! Vitamin C is another antioxidant that strengthens the immune system. It's vital to the growth and repair of skin, blood vessels, ligaments, and tendons. It is also involved with healing wounds and forming scar tissue.

Plus, vitamin C is important for the formation of collagen, which holds your body's cells together. And, it plays an important role in maintaining oral and eye health.

Many fruits are excellent sources of vitamin C, including:

- Cantaloupe
- Citrus fruits
- Kiwi
- Mango
- Guava

- Papaya
- Pineapple
- Berries
- Watermelon

You can get vitamin C from vegetables too, like cruciferous veggies (broccoli, cauliflower, and Brussels sprouts), peppers, leafy greens, potatoes, tomatoes, and squash.

Vitamin E

The third antioxidant we're concerned about is vitamin E. This nutrient helps widen blood vessels and keeps blood from clotting inside them. Foods that are high in vitamin E will also protect your skin from ultraviolet light, which is a major cause of free radical formation in the body.

Excellent sources of vitamin E include:

- Spinach
- Chard
- Turnip greens
- Mustard greens
- Cayenne pepper

- Asparagus
- Bell peppers
- Eggs
- Nuts and seeds
- Meats
- Olive oil
- Whole grains

Nutrition

Eating a well-balanced diet should provide essential nutrients, but there are some situations that definitely call for adding in supplements. When your diet isn't properly balanced, it doesn't contain adequate amounts of certain nutrients. In this case, supplements may be absolutely necessary.

In order for our body to use food to repair and create cells and tissues, it needs the proper tools. The following nutrients are extremely important to maintain a healthy body. And just like the majority of antioxidant sources, these nutrients are often found in abundance in plant-sourced foods.

Magnesium is not only an essential nutrient, but is responsible for a vast variety of healthy body functions. It also is the most deficient mineral in the Standard American Diet because it can be difficult to meet the daily requirements just from food. Less than 30% of U.S. adults consume the Recommended Daily Allowance of magnesium. And nearly 20% get only half of the magnesium they need daily to remain healthy.

To make sure you get enough magnesium in your diet, eat plenty of whole grains, legumes, vegetables, nuts, seeds, and seafood.

Calcium is the most abundant mineral in your body. It is responsible for strong teeth and bones, as well as proper function of blood vessels, nerve communication, and muscles. Many Americans suffer from a deficiency in calcium. We lose calcium each day through our skin, nails, hair, sweat, and waste.

To make sure you get enough calcium in your diet, make sure you consume dairy products, broccoli, kale, chinese cabbage, and salmon regularly. Depending on your diet and age, your doctor might recommend a calcium supplement.

Iron is important for the production of hemoglobin (found in red blood cells) and myoglobin (found in muscles). These proteins carry and store oxygen throughout the body. When you don't have enough iron in your body you feel tired, weak, and unable to focus. Few people ever have too much iron in the body, but this rare condition is toxic.

Excellent sources of iron include red meat, liver, egg yolks, leafy green veggies, dried fruits, shellfish, beans, lentils, and artichokes. Pairing iron-rich foods with vitamin C-rich foods will help your body absorb the iron better.

Iron deficiency can affect anyone, but it is extremely common among women of childbearing age. Your chiropractor can help you adjust your diet or recommend an iron supplement when necessary.

Vitamin D helps our bodies in the absorption of calcium. Vitamin D also increases bone density and helps prevent bone fractures. Plus, calcium helps regulate the immune system and protects against some types of cancer.

Humans can synthesize their own vitamin D – all it takes is a little sunshine. If you spend a little time in the sun each day, it is unlikely you will be deficient in vitamin D.

People in warm climates rarely have vitamin D problems – it's our neighbors to the north who tend to hibernate through cold, cloudy winters who suffer. If you live far north of the equator, all it really takes is exposing your skin to the sun for about 20 minutes per day (or a little bit longer for older or dark-skinned people) prior to applying sunscreen on most summer days. If you do this, your body will probably synthesize enough vitamin D to last the whole year.

Folic acid is a B vitamin. It helps your body make new cells, repair DNA, and prevent alzheimer's, anemia, and some forms of cancer.

It is extremely important for pregnant women to get enough folic acid not only while pregnant, but prior to pregnancy too. One of the first stages of pregnancy includes the development of the brain and spinal cord, so getting enough folic acid during this process is vital to proper fetal development. Insufficient folic acid has been linked to birth defects including spina bifida and anencephaly.

Veggies and citrus fruits are the best sources of folic acid. Eat plenty of dark leafy greens, asparagus, broccoli, beans, citrus fruits, peas, lentils, avocado, seeds and nuts, carrots, and squash.

Eating a healthy, well-balanced diet can provide you with a strong, energetic, efficient, healthy body. The best way to know if you are getting all the elements that make up a fully functioning healthy body is to discuss your diet with your chiropractor or health care professional. Together, you can ensure that you are providing the optimum fuel to your body.

Your body is designed to heal itself. The nervous system is what controls your immune system. If you're run down, your body is less able to cope with germs and infections. This is when we tend to experience illness or pain. If your nervous system is strong and healthy, your body can deal with injuries and germs better. Chiropractic care focuses on helping you maintain a strong and healthy nervous system, resulting in a healthy body and lifestyle.

CHAPTER 9

Getting Back to the Basics of Wellness

For a moment, think back to when you were a kid. Chances are that back in elementary school, you had boundless energy. The days were long but it didn't matter - you could probably run around the neighborhood with your friends with hardly a thought of food, pain, or fatigue.

Now maybe you have kids or grandkids, and you watch them go at playtime for hours without a pause – and it's exhausting! We joke about bottling all that energy. We get nostalgic about feeling limitless and free, but not enough of us know that there really is a way to regain some of those powerful feelings again.

Wellness is very personal and means different things to different people in terms of preferences and outcomes.

- If you have debilitating back pain, you might feel powerful again if you could get through the day without taking prescription painkillers and suffering through their side effects.
- If your arthritis restricts your daily physical activities, you might feel powerful again if you could go for a hike again, or knit another afghan without it resulting in days of excruciating joint pain.
- If you suffer from peripheral neuropathy, you might feel powerful again if you could regain sensation in your fingertips again and take up the activities and hobbies you left behind years ago.

Getting older isn't for sissies – but remember that we are lucky to have made it this far!

So what will it take for you to feel energetic and powerful again? There is no correct blanket answer to that question. Every person presents their own set of symptoms, conditions, and preferences. Plus, each person has their own set of goals that will make them feel healthy and happy. All of that makes it complicated to prescribe a roadmap to wellness.

As we discussed in prior chapters, we offer several healing modalities in our office that patients with chronic pain find to be beneficial. Vibration, low-light laser therapy, and electro therapy are a few important resources that many of our patients use every day. We also counsel our patients about the importance of eating a well-balanced diet.

Good nutrition should be considered the cornerstone of any wellness plan. The food you use to fuel your body will make a huge difference when your cells need to repair and regenerate themselves. We promote a diet that's big on unprocessed foods, fruits, vegetables, whole grains, and lean protein. Eating like this gives your body the vitamins, minerals, and antioxidants it needs to stay strong and healthy.

What Else Can I Do to Feel Well?

At the heart of our practice is a busy wellness clinic that offers chiropractic. We strongly believe in the power of a strong, aligned spine that supports a healthy central nervous system. Keeping the spine aligned is achieved through gentle, routine chiropractic adjustments. For most of our patients, one adjustment a week works great. But patients recovering from an accident, illness, infection, or injury sometimes require more frequent adjustments for a period of time.

Regular chiropractic adjustments can not only improve the health of your spine and nervous system, but they can also:

- Improve mood
- Improve sleep
- Increase energy
- Decrease pain
- Boost flexibility and mobility
- Stop recurring headaches

One of the most important things chiropractic adjustments do is boost the immune system. This is accomplished by clearing the neural pathways so that the central nervous system can communicate effectively with the immune system (and every other system in your body). This communication is hindered when the spine experiences subluxations, which are misalignments along the spinal column. When the nervous system's pathways are cleared, the effects can be quite powerful:

- Decrease in colds, flu, and other contagious illnesses
- Slash the symptoms of asthma and allergies
- Result in fewer hospital admissions

Unfortunately, most people only think to go to the chiropractor if their back hurts. But we can do so much more together than just fix back pain!

What Does Chiropractic Do for Peripheral Neuropathy?

As you may recall, the treatment modalities we already discussed for peripheral neuropathy were all about rebuilding nerves, growing blood vessels, and improving muscle function. Well chiropractic is all about clearing the way for the nervous system to do its job right. So when your brain can tell those tiny nerve endings that it's time to regrow, all those other efforts we talked about are far more likely to be successful.

In addition to fostering the regrowth of damaged nerves, chiropractic can also un-pinch nerves. A pinched nerve can cause numbness and pain, just like peripheral neuropathy. Getting the bones back into their proper places takes pressure off nerves, alleviates pain, and promotes a healthy, active lifestyle. It also gets the joint in the hands, feet or both moving better if affected by neuropathy.

What Should I Do if I Suspect That I Have Peripheral Neuropathy?

The National Institutes of Neurological Disorders and Stroke says that peripheral neuropathy affects roughly 24 million Americans. It's a very common condition among people in certain populations, such as diabetics, cancer patients, and those taking statin medications to lower their cholesterol. Therefore, it's important to know that if you do have peripheral neuropathy, you are certainly not alone.

While the early stages of the symptoms may seem to be just minor irritations, early diagnosis of peripheral neuropathy can prevent the condition from becoming worse. Talk to your doctor right away to diagnose and determine the cause of your peripheral neuropathy. There could be ways to change your medical treatment plan that can reduce your symptoms.

We also strongly recommend visiting a chiropractor as soon as you can. They may be able to offer you a variety of treatments that can reduce or even eliminate the pain, numbness, and tingling associated with PN. There is no reason to wait until the problem becomes worse – as soon as you suspect that something is wrong, seek professional help. It's the best way to ensure your health and wellness for many years to come.

CHAPTER 10

Would I Recommend This To My Friends & Family?

If I would not recommend this to my friends of family, I sure would not recommend it to any of my patients. In fact, I recommended the natural treatment protocol I discuss throughout this book for my own mother. She was involved in a bad car accident at the young age of 14. At the time of impact, a can opener stabbed my mother in her right leg, which ended up causing such severe infection that her leg had to be amputated. Since then, she has been dealing with severe nerve pain.

Upon performing a sensory exam in my office, she discovered just how much sensory loss she actually was experiencing in both her left leg, as well as her residual leg (right leg, amputated from right above her knee). Her left leg demonstrated 60% sensory loss and her right leg (stump/residual limb) demonstrated 94.29% sensory loss. Following this exam, she was provided with my recommendations for a natural treatment protocol. The most important part about the recommendations that I provided her was that in order to see best results she would need to be all-in and follow the treatment plan fully. Being the strong-willed woman that she is, I had full confidence in her ability to follow through. If I am being honest, and she will tell you herself, she had her doubts. Like most patients that get to this point after years of living with it and have had such a traumatic onset of symptoms, she had every right to doubt the process. She's been through almost every test you can think of and has even been to Mayo Clinic in search of answers. Unfortunately, even the Mayo Clinic was unable to provide her with any options other than the traditional methods of medications and surgery, and they told her that she would have to deal with it for the rest of her life. Hope had been lost and she was simply living with the pain, managing it as best as she could.

Within the first few weeks of the program, I received a call from my mother and she quickly became emotional over the phone as she informed me that she could now feel tingling in her left ankle. At first, she thought there was no way this was happening and it must be "in her head," so she ignored it and didn't bother telling me about the first time it happened. Then, it became apparent that it was happening more often and she could feel more tingling, which she could not feel before starting the program.

Fast forward to her exam after a short three months; I performed a follow up sensory exam to track and assess her results. The results were outstanding. In the right residual limb, it showed a 41.47% sensory loss, resulting in a 56.1% improvement from the initial exam. Her left leg showed a 2.86% sensory loss, resulting in a 95.23% improvement from the initial exam. While this is very encouraging, please note that every person heals differently and at different rates.

Additionally, we use thermal imaging to assess for loss of circulation as another part of our exam process and data collection for each case. On her initial exam, the heat represented in red stopped just below the knee on her left leg indicating poor blood supply and circulation in that left leg. At the end of the short three months, her leg was fully red and she no longer felt coldness in her left foot. She went on to say: "After 34 years of living with nerve damage due to a traumatic leg injury, I have regained sensation. I am truly amazed at how the body has the ability to heal and regenerate even after decades of damage. My toenails have regained color under the nail beds and I no longer have to wear a knee length sock for warmth."

To add to this amazing healing story, she went in to her doctor for Ankle Brachial Index (ABI) testing after I had performed her progress examination at the three month mark of her undergoing our treatment program. The ABI test is a test used to diagnose peripheral arterial disease and the lack of blood flow by comparing her upper extremities with the lower extremities. A typical normal range is within 1.0-1.4. In 2016, she had the ABI test performed and was considered in the moderate to severe category with the posterior tibial artery with ABI of 0.54, which has the prognosis of worsening over time. She had another test scheduled in 2021 and I remember telling my mother that I am excited to see what the results are for the ABI test, because I think they are going to be shocked by what they find since she had been working with me to reverse her condition. The results of the 2021 ABI test were remarkable. She was now considered in the normal range and her new ABI was 1.09. After listening to a voicemail that was sent to my mother's phone by the examining office, it was clear that she had stunned them. They stated that the results "look good, and they actually look better and had improved since last time." They didn't have an explanation of why, but she was beyond excited for these results.

The email stated:

"Tracy,

As you can see below with the test results, your circulation appears to have improved from the moderate-severe category of Peripheral Arterial Disease with the Posterior Tibial Artery to the normal range. Typically, over time we see the opposite – but for you your blood flow appears to have improved from 2016 until recently."

It's moments like these that are truly priceless because she had been one of many patients that was told that she would not be able to do anything to reverse her condition and that she would have to live with it, which meant that she might eventually lose her one and only good leg.

You may be thinking this is just one story from one person and these results are just an impressive fluke. I assure you that there are thousands of patients nationwide seeing similar results on a daily basis. When the medical world says it cannot be done, the natural world says: "yes it can." Keep reading into the next chapter to hear more testimonials about the incredible healing potential of the body that demonstrates that our bodies are resilient and there really can be hope for neuropathy.

CHAPTER 11

Testimonials

"Within 90 days, the sensory loss in my feet improved by 25% in one foot and 32% in the other foot. I was also going through chemo while on this program and still got optimal results. I definitely would recommend this program for anyone who is struggling with sensory loss so they can get their life back. I am excited about the improvement I have made in only 90 days. This program changed my life."

–Laura C.

"After 31 visits, I was 90-95% cured & I am very fortunate that I came in for care."

–Bill M.

"After only 2 treatments I was able to sleep at night without socks which had been one of my big problems because my feet had been so cold."

–Mickey W.

"I was taking pain medication every day, after 12 visits I stopped taking pain medication. I had no symptoms at night and I did not need sleeping aids anymore. I am extremely happy with my choice to begin the program."

–Rosanna V.

"I have gone from 44% sensory loss down to 15% sensory loss halfway through the program. I'm getting better and I feel a whole lot better."

–Kim M.

"I saw an ad for neuropathy which intrigued me because I was developing neuropathy in my feet and legs. I saw my podiatrist and he confirmed that I have neuropathy. So, I decided to try the program;

I had always had trouble with my legs particularly. I could not sleep at night because my legs bothered me so much – in less than 2 weeks I was beginning to sleep through the night!"

–Bob B.

"The pain in my feet was so severe, I could barely walk by the end of the day. After starting the neuropathy program, I have noticed that the pain in my feet is almost gone, in just 7 weeks."

–Harold D.

"I came here because of the numbness in my feet, it was all over the top and bottom of my feet as well as my toes. I've been on the program awhile now and all I have is a little bit of numbness so it is definitely working. I would encourage anyone to come here and visit with them. I have been very happy and I believe their maintenance program will help me as well!"

–Matt B.

"Over 5 years ago, I was told by a well-respected neurologist that "nothing can be done other than take B12 and be careful not to fall". I heard about this program at a local rotary meeting, thought I would give it a try...fully expecting a similar situation because of my age. To my surprise after testing, I knew there was potential that I could really get some help. I am now in my 8th week of therapy and the results have been amazing. No longer have tingling sensation or pain."

–Burnell S.

"I have been coming in for treatment for about a week and half now. Since then I have lost nine pounds sticking to the nutrition plan. I have such bad feet problems, back pain, neck pain, and hand pain that's why I decided to come...since I've been coming, I have already seen quite a bit of difference in this short amount of time. I can't believe the progress I've had in such a short amount of time."

–Ann R.

"My feet have been dead for quite some time. Two different times in my pick-up, I couldn't feel my accelerator. We started the treatment and about 3-4 weeks into the program, after beginning the home treatment...I could feel the carpet when I was walking and that was the first time I had done that in quite some time."

–Mark O.

"I was having pretty bad neuropathy and it was continuing to get worse after seeing medical doctors, they were just giving me some pain pills and vitamin B12 shots. I decided I needed to do something better & be proactive. This will be my third week and between all the treatments they do here, I am already improving – I'm down to one incident a week and I was having 5-6 incidents a day."

–Kelly C.

"Neuropathy was effecting my life pretty bad for almost a year now, to the point where I was in pain most of the time. Since I've been coming here for 3 or 4 sessions now, I have already noticed a lot of difference and I am already feeling a lot better.

–Jesse R.

"I came here very apprehensive. I have been coming only a few weeks now and I have already regained so much strength in my left leg which was the problem. I barely use my cane at all now – just for a little security. I just can't believe how well I am doing after only being treated for a short amount of time!"

–Dorothy C.

"I have suffered from neuropathy for at least three years, I have been completing treatment here and it has already been successful. I can sleep at night without my feet burning and hurting!"

–Betty P.

"I came to here because I have neuropathy and it is effecting my golf game. I have been coming about five weeks and I can already tell some improvement in the bottom of my feet."

–Gary C.

"I am relatively new to the program, this is only my third visit. I have already gone from a pain level of 8 to a pain level of 2!"

– Kim N.

"I have been coming about 6 weeks. When I came in, I had severe pain all the way from my hip down to my big toe. As of today, I am able to wiggle my big toe and I have feeling in it! I have NO more pain in my hips or legs. Overall, my time spent here has been well worthwhile! I must say that the staff has been very professional, helpful, and encouraging."

–Nell M.

"I am in my 3rd week of my treatment, when I came in, my left foot was killing me and my right foot was not far behind it. I was asked to rate my pain on a level of 1 – 10 during my consultation and I have been at a level 10 for about three or four months now. My pain level now is nearly gone completely."

–James F.

"I came here after seeing the ad in the paper, I decided to come in because of my neuropathy being so bad. It took a little bit of work but everything they have done here for me has been very great. The staff here is very nice which helps a lot when coming in for treatment."

–Everisto M.

Bibliography

1. https://www.commonwealthfund.
    org/publications/fund-reports/2021/
    aug/mirror-mirror-2021-reflecting-
    poorly#:~:text=Health%20Care%20
    System%20Performance%20
    Rankings&text=The%20U.S.%20ranks%20
    %2311%20%E2%80%94%20last,above%20
    it%2C%20Switzerland%20and%20Canada.

2. Go AS, Mozaffarian D, Roger VL, Benjamin EJ,
    Berry JD, Borden WB, Bravata DM, Dai S, Ford
    ES, Fox CS, Franco S, Fullerton HJ, Gillespie C,
    Hailpern SM, Heit JA, Howard VJ, Huffman MD,
    Kissela BM, Kittner SJ, Lackland DT, Lichtman
    JH, Lisabeth LD, Magid D, Marcus GM, Marelli
    A, Matchar DB, McGuire DK, Mohler ER, Moy

CS, Mussolino ME, Nichol G, Paynter NP, Schreiner PJ, Sorlie PD, Stein J, Turan TN, Virani SS, Wong ND, Woo D, Turner MB; on behalf of the American Heart Association Statistics Committee and Stroke Statistics Subcommittee. Heart disease and stroke statistics—2013 update: a report from the American Heart Association.Circulation.2013;127:e6-e245.

3. Masters, Ryan, PhD. News. Columbia University Mailman School of Public Health. "Obesity Kills More Americans Than Previously Thought". N.p., 15 Aug. 2013.

4. Kochanek KD, Xu JQ, Murphy SL, Miniño AM, Kung HC. Deaths: final data for 2009. Adobe PDF file [PDF-2M] National vital statistics reports. 2011; 60(3).

5. Heidenreich PA, Trogdon JG, Khavjou OA, et al. Forecasting the future of cardiovascular disease in the United States: a policy statement from the American Heart Association. Circulation. 2011;123:933-44. Epub 2011 Jan 24.

6. Go AS, Mozaffarian D, Roger VL, Benjamin EJ, Berry JD, Borden WB, Bravata DM, Dai S, Ford ES, Fox CS, Franco S, Fullerton HJ, Gillespie C, Hailpern SM, Heit JA, Howard VJ, Huffman MD, Kissela BM, Kittner SJ, Lackland DT, Lichtman JH, Lisabeth LD, Magid D, Marcus GM, Marelli A, Matchar DB, McGuire DK, Mohler ER, Moy CS, Mussolino ME, Nichol G, Paynter NP, Schreiner PJ, Sorlie PD, Stein J, Turan TN, Virani SS, Wong ND, Woo D, Turner MB; on behalf of the American Heart Association Statistics Committee and Stroke Statistics Subcommittee. Heart disease and stroke statistics—2013 update: a report from the American Heart Association. Circulation.2013;127:e6-e245.

7. Go AS, Mozaffarian D, Roger VL, Benjamin EJ, Berry JD, Borden WB, Bravata DM, Dai S, Ford ES, Fox CS, Franco S, Fullerton HJ, Gillespie C, Hailpern SM, Heit JA, Howard VJ, Huffman MD, Kissela BM, Kittner SJ, Lackland DT, Lichtman JH, Lisabeth LD, Magid D, Marcus GM, Marelli A, Matchar DB, McGuire

DK, Mohler ER, Moy CS, Mussolino ME, Nichol G, Paynter NP, Schreiner PJ, Sorlie PD, Stein J, Turan TN, Virani SS, Wong ND, Woo D, Turner MB; on behalf of the American Heart Association Statistics Committee and Stroke Statistics Subcommittee. Heart disease and stroke statistics—2013 update: a report from the American Heart Association. Circulation.2013;127:e6-e245.

8. American Cancer Society. Cancer Facts & Figures 2013. Atlanta: American Cancer Society; 2013.

9. "Diabetes Statistics." Diabetes Basics. American Diabetes Association, 2013.

10. "Osteoporosis." NIHSeniorHealth.

11. Chris L. Peterson, Rachel Burton. *The U.S. Health Care Spending*. 2008.

12. Kane, Jason. "Health Costs: How the U.S. Compares With Other Countries." PBS. PBS, 22 Oct. 2012. Web.

13. "News Release." *USDA Celebrates National Farmers Market Week*, August 4-10. United

States Department of Agriculture, 5 Aug. 2013. Web. 02 Aug. 2015. <http://www.usda. gov/wps/portal/usda/usdahome?contentid= 2013%2F08%2F0155.xml>.

14. "Office of Public and Intergovernmental Affairs." News Releases -. VA Office of Public and Intergovernmental Affairs, 25 Feb. 2014. Web. 02 Aug. 2015. <http://www.va.gov/opa/ pressrel/pressrelease.cfm?id=2529>.

15. Eisenberg, DM, Kessler, RC, et al. New England Journal Medicine, "Unconventional Medicine in the United States -- Prevalence, Costs, and Patterns of Use." 1993.

16. Swift, Art. "Half of Americans Take Vitamins Regularly." Gallup.com. N.p., 19 Dec. 2013. Web. 02 Aug. 2015. <http://www.gallup. com/poll/166541/half-americans-vitamins- regularly.aspx>.

17. Who Killed Health Care?: America's $2 Trillion Medical Problem - and the Consumer-Driven Cure, Regina Herzlinger, 2007.

18.   Mayo Clinic Staff. "Peripheral Neuropathy."
       Causes. Mayo Clinic, 04 Dec. 2014. Web.
       22 July 2015. http://www.mayoclinic.org/
       diseases-conditions/peripheral-neuropathy/
       basics/causes/CON-20019948.

19.   "The ReBuilder® Stops Pain While Treating
       Your Nerves - at Home." Safe, Effective
       Neuropathy Treatment. Web. 25 July 2015.
       <http://www.rebuildermedical.com/>.

20.   "Frequently Asked Questions." Frequently
       Asked Questions. Web. 25 July 2015. <http://
       www.rebuildermedical.com/frequently-
       asked-questions.php#chemo>.

21.   Loghmani MT, Warden SJ. "Instrument-
       assisted cross-fiber massage accelerates
       knee ligament healing." Journal of
       Orthopaedic Sports Physical Therapy. 2009.

22.   LeBauer A, Brtalik R, Stowe K. "The effect of
       myofascial release (MFR) on an adult with
       idiopathic scoliosis." Journal of Bodywork
       and Movement Therapies. 2008.

23. J Bodyw Mov Ther. 2013 Oct;17(4):518-22. doi: 10.1016/j.jbmt.2013.03.001. Epub 2013 Apr 30. http://www.ncbi.nlm.nih.gov/pubmed/24139013.

24. "Why Use VibePlate for Vibration Therapy, Vibration Traning, & Vibration Exercise." Why Use VibePlate for Vibration Therapy, Vibration Traning, & Vibration Exercise. N.p., n.d. Web. 26 July 2015. <http://www.vibeplate.net/why-vibeplate>.

25. MedlinePlus (June 7, 2012). U.S. National Library of Medicine. Medline Plus Trusted Health Information for You. Beta-carotene. Retrieved from www.nlm.nih.gov/medlineplus/druginfo/natural/999.html.

26. LL Magnetic Clay Inc.(1996-2010). Ancient Minerals:.Need More Magnesium? 10 Signs to Watch For. Retrieved from: www.ancient-minerals.com/magnesium-deficiency/need-more/.

27. WebMD.(2005–2012). Weight Loss & Diet Plans. Top 10 Iron-Rich Foods. Retrieved from:

www.webmd.com/diet/features/top-10-iron-rich-foods.

28. More, J. (Sept. 2008). The British Dietetic Association. Vitamin D- The Unique Vitamin. Retrieved from: www.bda.uk.com/foodfacts/VitaminD.pdf.

29. Ferreira, Leonor Mateus. "Chiropractic Care May Help Control Peripheral Neuropathy in Diabetics." Diabetes News Journal. N.p., 16 Mar. 2015. Web. 27 July 2015. <http://diabetesnewsjournal.com/2015/03/17/chiropractic-care-may-help-control-peripheral-neuropathy-in-diabetics/>.

30. https://my.clevelandclinic.org/health/diagnostics/17840-ankle-brachial-index-abi#:~:text=Results%20and%20Follow%2DUp,-What%20do%20the&text=An%20ABI%20ratio%20between%201.0,means%20you%20have%20moderate%20PAD.

Notes

Notes

Notes

Notes

Notes

Notes

Notes

CPSIA information can be obtained
at www.ICGtesting.com
Printed in the USA
BVHW081433020522
635664BV00006B/23

9 781737 996163